Wall Pilates Workouts

The Ultimate 30-Day Challenge for Flexibility, Balance,

and Muscle Strength | Reshape Your Body with 3 Plans Included

PATRICIA VALE

TABLE OF CONTENTS

INTRODUCTION

Wall Pilates is a type of workout in which the body is supported and guided through various exercises by a wall. Individuals may improve their posture, boost their strength and flexibility, and establish a better mind-body connection by using the wall as a tool. Wall Pilates is a low-impact workout that is suitable for people of all fitness levels, from beginners to expert athletes.

One of the most important advantages of wall Pilates is that it helps enhance posture. Many people spend a lot of time sitting at a desk or bent over a computer, which can contribute to bad posture and back discomfort. Individuals may strengthen their core and back muscles by including wall Pilates into their workout program, which can improve their posture and lessen the chance of back problems.

Another advantage of wall Pilates is that it can help you gain strength and flexibility. Individuals can target certain muscle areas and increase their overall strength by using the wall as added resistance. Furthermore, wall Pilates stretching exercises can assist increase flexibility, which can lower the chance of injury and enhance overall sports performance.

Wall Pilates may also be a good kind of exercise for people who want to reduce weight or tone their body. Strength and aerobic activities combined can help burn calories and build lean muscle mass, improving overall body composition. Furthermore, concentrating on good breathing methods can help reduce stress and increase general well-being.

Overall, wall Pilates is a beneficial kind of training for people of all fitness levels. Wall Pilates may deliver a full-body exercise that targets various muscle groups and increases overall fitness, whether you're a novice or an established athlete.

However, to properly grasp the efficiency of wall Pilates, it is necessary to first comprehend the unique exercises and strategies utilized in this type of exercise. Some examples of wall Pilates exercises and how they might help the body are as follows:

1. Wall Plank: This exercise is identical to a standard plank, however it is supported by the wall. Individuals may develop their core and back muscles by activating the core and keeping the plank position, improving posture and lowering the risk of back injury.

2. Wall Sit: Similar to a squat, this exercise includes leaning against a wall with your legs sitting. Individuals may develop their leg

muscles and enhance general lower body strength by keeping the position.

3. Wall Roll Down: In this workout, the spine is rolled down the wall one vertebrae at a time. Individuals can enhance spine flexibility and lessen the risk of back discomfort by activating the core and focusing on good breathing.

4. Wall Squat: Similar to a wall sit, this exercise includes resting against a wall with the legs in a squat posture. Individuals can increase their total body composition and lower body strength by keeping the position and exercising the leg muscles.

5. Wall Push-Up: This exercise is similar to a typical push-up, except it is supported by a wall. Individuals may increase their general fitness and upper body strength by working the chest, arms, and core muscles.

Individuals may accomplish a full-body workout that targets several muscle groups and enhances overall health by adding these and other movements into their wall Pilates regimen. However, like with any kind of exercise, wall Pilates must be executed correctly in order to be effective and safe.

Individuals may enhance the efficiency of their wall Pilates exercises by practicing perfect technique and form, in addition to training with a trained instructor. This involves maintaining good posture, using the core muscles, and breathing properly. Starting with the fundamentals and progressively increasing the difficulty and intensity of the workouts over time is critical.

Consistency is another aspect that might influence the effectiveness of wall Pilates. It is critical to constantly execute, as with any sort of exercise.

To get improvements, perform wall Pilates routines. The 30-day training plan presented in "Wall Pilates Workouts: A Proven 30-Day Wall Pilates Plan to Gain Tone, Strength, and Reshape Your Body" is an excellent approach to maintain consistency and motivation. This plan contains posture and core routine exercises, balance routine activities, and flexibility and abs strengthen regular exercises, all of which are meant to take only a few minutes each day to complete. This makes it simple to include wall Pilates into even the most hectic of schedules.

Another advantage of wall Pilates is that it may help you improve your balance and stability. Individuals can undertake workouts that test their balance and stability by utilizing the wall as a tool, which can enhance overall sports performance and lessen the chance of falls and accidents. Wall Pilates is also a good alternative for people who have balance concerns or want to improve their balance and coordination.

Wall Pilates gives mental advantages in addition to physical benefits. Wall Pilates can help relieve stress and anxiety and enhance general mental well-being by emphasizing appropriate breathing methods and mind-body connection. This can contribute to increased attention, better sleep, and a general sense of well-being.

It is vital to remember that individual outcomes may differ when it comes to the effectiveness of wall Pilates. Wall Pilates outcomes can be influenced by factors such as general fitness level, consistency, and commitment to good technique and form. However, many people have found success with this type of training and have met their fitness objectives in as little as 30 days.

To summarize, wall Pilates is a distinct and efficient kind of exercise that may bring several benefits to people of all fitness levels. Individuals may enhance their posture, strength and flexibility, balance and stability, and attain their fitness objectives by including wall Pilates into their workout program. Wall Pilates may be a terrific addition to any training regimen if done correctly, consistently, and with desire. So why not give it a go and see what it can do for you?

CHAPTER 1: GETTING STARTED

Wall Pilates is a unique and effective kind of exercise that may bring several advantages to people of all fitness levels. But, before you begin a wall Pilates program, you need know what you'll need and how to prepare for your exercises. The following is a summary of what is needed:

A wall

The most significant piece of equipment need for wall Pilates is, of course, a wall. Look for a strong wall with adequate room to fit your body in various postures. The wall should ideally be smooth and devoid of any sharp or projecting things.

Comfortable Clothing

When it comes to wall Pilates clothes, comfort is essential. Look for clothing that is breathable, flexible, and allows you to move freely. Clothing that is overly tight or restricting might inhibit movement and reduce the efficacy of your activities.

A Mat

While wall Pilates is mostly done with the wall as a tool, a mat can be useful for giving extra cushioning and support during floor movements. Look for a thick and comfy mat that is also easy to clean and move.

Correct Footwear

While wall Pilates may be done barefoot, some people choose to use shoes for extra support and stability. Look for shoes that are flexible, comfy, and have a good grip on the floor.

Bottle of Water

It is critical to stay hydrated during your wall Pilates sessions in order to retain energy and attention. Bring a water bottle to your workouts and sip often throughout the session.

Towel

Sweating is an expected byproduct of any workout, even wall Pilates. Bring a towel to your exercises to help you dry off and avoid sliding.

Attitude of Positivity

Finally, a happy mindset is one of the most vital things you'll need for wall Pilates. Approach your workouts with an open mind and the desire to learn and grow. Celebrate minor successes and progress, and don't be disheartened if you run across difficulties.

You'll be ready to begin your road towards a stronger, healthier body if you collect these tools and prepare for your wall Pilates sessions. But, before we get started, it's necessary to grasp the importance of breathing in wall Pilates.

Proper breathing is an important part of wall Pilates and is required to get the most out of your exercises. Breathing is utilized in wall Pilates to stimulate core muscles, enhance posture, and boost attention and relaxation. Proper breathing can also aid in injury prevention and stress reduction.

Focus on breathing in through your nose and out through your mouth when practicing wall Pilates. Deeply inhale to extend your ribcage, then fully exhale to clench your abs. Focus on drawing your belly button towards your spine and using your core muscles as you exhale. This will aid in the activation of the deep abdominal muscles and the improvement of posture.

You'll be able to enhance the efficacy of each exercise and reach your fitness objectives faster if you incorporate appropriate breathing methods into your wall Pilates routines. So, take the time to practice appropriate breathing and prepare for your wall Pilates exercises, and prepare to see results in as little as 30 days.

Now that you know what you'll need and how to prepare for your wall Pilates workouts, it's time to get started on the exercises. In the next chapter, we'll look at several wall Pilates exercises that may help you gain strength, enhance flexibility, and improve your overall fitness.

CHAPTER 2: IMPORTANCE OF BREATHING

Proper breathing is an important part of wall Pilates and may have a significant impact on the efficiency of your workouts. Breathing is utilized in wall Pilates to stimulate core muscles, enhance posture, and boost attention and relaxation. Proper breathing can also aid in injury prevention and stress reduction.

The Breathing Process in Wall Pilates

Breathing is employed in wall Pilates to engage the core muscles and activate the deep abdominal muscles, which are essential for maintaining appropriate posture and alignment. By concentrating on good breathing methods, you may increase the efficiency of each activity and reach your fitness objectives more quickly.

Proper breathing also aids in stress reduction and relaxation, which is beneficial to both mental and physical health. You may minimize stress and anxiety and enhance your general feeling of well-being by employing breathing exercises to concentrate your attention and release tension.

2.1: Wall Pilates Breathing Techniques

In wall Pilates, numerous breathing methods are often employed, including:

Breathing Diaphragmatically

Diaphragmatic breathing is inhaling deeply through the nose, enabling the air to fill the lungs and expand the ribcage, and then fully expelling through the mouth while clenching the abs. This approach aids in the activation of deep abdominal muscles and the improvement of posture.

Breathing through the ribcage

Ribcage breathing is concentrating on the expansion and contraction of the ribcage with each breath. Inhale deeply while focusing on extending the ribcage, then exhale fully while contracting the abs and returning the ribcage back to its original position.

Counted breathing

Counted breathing consists of inhaling for a certain number of counts and then exhaling for the same number of counts. For example, you could inhale for four counts, hold for four counts, then exhale for four counts. This approach aids in the regulation of breathing and the promotion of relaxation.

2.2: Including Breathing Exercises in Your Wall Pilates Workouts

Including correct breathing practices in your wall design Pilates routines are required for the greatest outcomes. You may boost the efficacy of each workout and accomplish your fitness objectives faster by concentrating on appropriate breathing and using the core muscles.

Here are a few wall Pilates routines that integrate breathing techniques:

Diaphragmatic Breathing on the Wall

Stand with your back to the wall and gently slide down until your knees are at a 90-degree angle to do a wall sit with diaphragmatic breathing. Maintain this position by breathing deeply through your nostrils and stretching your ribcage. Then, while clenching your abs, thoroughly exhale through your lips. This exercise will aid in the activation of the deep abdominal muscles and the improvement of posture.

Push-ups against the wall with ribcage breathing

To do a wall push-up with ribcage breathing, face the wall and position your hands shoulder-width apart on the wall. Lower your body slowly toward the wall while maintaining your abs engaged and your spine straight. As you push yourself back up, concentrate on breathing deeply and stretching your ribcage. Then fully exhale while clenching your abs. This exercise will aid in the activation of core muscles and the improvement of posture.

Roll-Down Wall with Counted Breathing

Stand with your back against the wall and steadily roll down through each vertebrae until your hands reach the floor to complete a wall roll-down with counted breathing. Inhale for four counts as you slide down. Hold for four counts, then exhale for four counts as you gently roll back up. This practice will help you control your breathing and relax.

You may increase your overall fitness and attain your objectives faster by including correct breathing methods into your wall Pilates sessions. Remember to keep appropriate technique and alignment in mind while you execute each exercise, and to listen to your body and modify as necessary.

2.3: The Advantages of Proper Breathing in Wall Pilates

In addition to increasing the efficacy of your exercises, good breathing methods in wall Pilates provide a variety of health and wellbeing advantages. Here are a some of the several advantages of correct breathing in wall Pilates:

- Improved Posture: perfect breathing in wall Pilates can assist improve posture and minimize tension on the back and neck by activating the core muscles and maintaining perfect alignment.

- Increased Flexibility: Deep breathing improves flexibility and range of motion by increasing blood flow and oxygen to the muscles.

- Stress Reduction: Concentrating on good breathing methods can help decrease stress and promote relaxation, both of which can enhance general mental and physical health.

- Improved attention: During your wall Pilates workouts, you may enhance your attention and concentration by focusing on your breath and utilizing your core muscles.

2.4: Tips for Improving Your Breathing Techniques in Wall Pilates

If you're new to wall Pilates or having trouble with correct breathing methods, here are a few pointers to help you:

- Collaborate with a Certified Instructor: A qualified wall Pilates teacher can advise you on optimal breathing methods and assist you in getting the most out of your exercises.

- Regular practice: Proper breathing methods in wall Pilates, like any talent, take consistent practice to perfect. Spend time focusing on your breathing throughout each workout, and experiment with incorporating breathing methods into your daily life.

- Focus on the Exhale: In wall Pilates, the exhale is frequently more crucial than the inhale. You may activate the core muscles and enhance posture by completely inhaling and contracting the abs.

- Pay Attention to Your Body: Because everyone's body is unique, it's critical to listen to your body and alter your breathing method as needed. If you experience pain or discomfort while exercising, stop and seek medical attention.

You may reach your fitness objectives and enhance your quality of life by including appropriate breathing methods into your wall Pilates routines and concentrating on the advantages of deep breathing for general health and wellness. In the next chapter, we'll look at several wall Pilates exercises that may help you gain strength, enhance flexibility, and improve your overall fitness.

CHAPTER 3: SAFETY TIPS

Safety Recommendations

While wall Pilates may be a terrific method to enhance your fitness and general health, each activity should be approached with caution. Here are some crucial safety precautions to remember when performing wall Pilates:

Warm-up and cool-down periods

It is critical to warm up and cool down appropriately before commencing any wall Pilates practice. This helps your muscles prepare for the activity and prevents injuries. Gentle stretching or aerobic activities like jumping jacks or walking in place might be included in a warm-up. More stretching or relaxation methods, such as deep breathing, might be used in a cool-down.

Correct Form and Alignment

Proper form and alignment are critical for avoiding injury and maximizing the benefits of your wall Pilates training. Here are some pointers to help you keep appropriate form and alignment:

Activate your core: Throughout the workout, your core muscles should be engaged. This protects your back and improves your posture.

Maintain a neutral spine position: Avoid arching your spine or rounding your back. Instead, keep your shoulders back and down and your chest open to maintain a neutral spine.

Maintain a relaxed stance: Relax your shoulders and keep them away from your ears. Avoid tensing or shrugging your shoulders.

Align your knees and ankles as follows: When completing leg workouts, ensure sure your knees and ankles are correctly aligned. Your knees should be squarely above your ankles, and your feet should face forward.

Using the Correct Equipment

A safe and effective wall Pilates workout requires the use of the correct equipment. Here are some pointers to remember:

Use a strong wall: Check that the wall you're utilizing is strong enough to sustain your weight. Use caution when utilizing walls with peeling paint or loose wallpaper.

Use a mat: A mat can assist cushion your joints and keep you from slipping.

Wear loose-fitting clothing: Wear clothing that provides a complete range of motion and is easy to move in. Avoid wearing clothes that is overly tight or constricting.

Paying Attention to Your Body

Listening to your body is essential for avoiding injury and overexertion. Here are some pointers to help you listen to your body:

Don't push yourself through pain: If you experience pain or discomfort while exercising, stop immediately and rest. If the discomfort persists, seek the advice of a medical expert.

Take pauses as needed: If you are weary or exhausted, stop and rest. Don't push yourself past your comfort zone.

Keep hydrated: To avoid dehydration, drink lots of water before, during, and after your workout.

You can assure a safe and productive wall Pilates practice by remembering these safety considerations. In the next chapter, we'll look at several wall Pilates exercises that may help you gain strength, enhance flexibility, and improve your overall fitness.

Specific Needs Modifications

If you have any special health problems or physical limits, you may modify your wall Pilates routines to guarantee safety and efficacy. Here are some instances of adaptations for special requirements:

Pregnancy: Pregnant women can do wall Pilates safely with few adjustments. Avoid laying on your back or exerting pressure on your abdomen, and instead focus on activities that develop pelvic stability and lower body strength.

If you have joint discomfort, avoid high-impact workouts and instead focus on low-impact exercises that are soft on the joints. Props such as cushions or blankets can also be used to cushion your joints during activities.

Osteoporosis: If you have osteoporosis, avoid workouts that require you to lean forward or twist your spine. Instead, concentrate on workouts that build balance and lower-body strength.

Common Errors to Avoid

Here are some frequent blunders to avoid when doing wall Pilates:

Holding your breath might induce stress and reduce the efficiency of the activity. Throughout each exercise, focus on breathing deeply and continuously.

Overarching the back: Overarching the back can cause lower back strain and damage. Maintain a neutral spine by using the core muscles.

Using momentum to finish an activity can impair its efficacy and raise the danger of injury. To get the most out of each workout, focus on controlled, deliberate movements.

You can assure a safe and efficient wall Pilates practice by avoiding these frequent errors and applying adaptations as needed. Always listen to your body, take pauses as required, and seek the advice of a healthcare expert if you have any concerns.

In the next chapter, we'll look at several wall Pilates exercises that can help you gain strength, enhance flexibility, and improve your overall fitness.

CHAPTER 4: WALL EXERCISES

Wall training is a form of exercise that involves various types of exercises suitable for both beginners and experienced individuals. It is essential to select exercises based on personal fitness levels, targeted muscle groups, and desired outcomes. The choice of exercises should be aligned with the purpose one intends to pursue with the workout. This is why it is necessary to pick exercises that best suit personal plans and needs.

This overview highlights some of the most popular wall training exercises. These exercises are grouped based on their type and the goals they aim to achieve with regular practice over time. The categorization allows individuals to choose exercises that align with their fitness objectives. For instance, exercises aimed at building endurance and strength will be different from those focused on flexibility and agility.

In summary, wall training exercises cater to a broad range of fitness levels, allowing individuals to choose exercises that align with their fitness goals. The categorization of exercises based on their type and fitness objectives simplifies the selection process, enabling individuals to pick exercises that best suit their plans and needs.

Wall Hamstring Stretch: involves lying on your back with your legs stretched up against a wall and your hips near the wall. Flex your feet and gently bring your toes closer to your shins to deepen the stretch. Hold this position for 30 to 60 seconds. This exercise primarily targets the hamstrings and can help improve flexibility and reduce muscle tension in the legs. It is important to perform this exercise with care and to stop immediately if you experience any pain or discomfort.

Wall Chest Stretch: stand facing away from a wall and put one hand on it at shoulder height. Turn your body away from the wall until you feel a stretch in your chest. Hold this for 30-60 seconds before switching sides. It targets the chest and shoulders, making it ideal for those who spend a lot of time sitting or hunching over a computer. It helps to improve posture, reduce the risk of injury in the shoulders, neck, and upper back. Care should be taken to stop if any pain or discomfort is felt, and medical advice sought if necessary.

Wall Calf Stretch: stand facing a wall and place your hands on it at shoulder height. Take a step back with one foot and press your heel into the floor, keeping your other leg straight. Hold for 30-60 seconds before switching sides. This exercise targets the calves and helps improve flexibility, reduce muscle tension, and prevent injury in the lower legs.

Wall Spine Stretch: lie on your back with legs up the wall and arms at shoulder height to the sides. Lower your knees to one side, while keeping your shoulders on the floor. Hold for 30-60 seconds before switching sides. This exercise targets the back and oblique muscles, helping to improve spinal mobility and flexibility.

Wall Pec Stretch: involves standing facing a wall and placing one hand on it at shoulder height. Rotate your body away from the wall until you feel a stretch in your chest. Hold this position for 30-60 seconds before switching sides. This exercise targets the chest and shoulders, helping to improve posture and reduce the risk of injury in the upper body. Care should be taken to stop if any pain or discomfort is felt.

Wall Lateral Stretch: involves standing facing a wall with your hands on it at shoulder height. Step back with one foot and rest your torso against the wall while keeping your hips square. Hold this position for 30-60 seconds before switching sides. This exercise targets the oblique and side body muscles, helping to improve spinal mobility and flexibility.

Wall Quadriceps Stretch: involves standing facing a wall and placing one hand on it for balance. Bend one knee and pull your foot towards your buttocks, gripping your ankle with your hand. Hold this position for 30-60 seconds before switching sides. This exercise targets the quadriceps, helping to improve flexibility, reduce muscle tension, and prevent injury in the legs. Care should be taken to stop if any pain or discomfort is felt, and medical advice sought if necessary.

Wall Figure Four Stretch: involves lying on your back with your feet up against a wall and your knees bent. Cross one ankle over the opposite knee and slide your foot down the wall until you feel a stretch in your hip. Hold this position for 30-60 seconds before switching sides. This exercise targets the hip muscles, helping to improve flexibility, reduce muscle tension, and prevent injury in the hips and lower back.

Wall Shoulder Stretch, stand facing a wall and place one hand on it at shoulder height. Slowly rotate your body away from the wall while keeping your arm straight. Hold this position for 30-60 seconds before switching sides. This exercise targets the shoulders and upper back, helping to improve flexibility, reduce muscle tension, and prevent injury in the upper body.

Wall Triceps Stretch: stand facing a wall and place one hand on it at shoulder height, with your palm facing down. Slowly lean against the wall while keeping your arm straight. Hold this position for 30-60 seconds before switching sides. This exercise targets the triceps muscles, helping to improve flexibility, reduce muscle tension, and prevent injury in the arms and shoulders. Care should be taken to stop if any pain or discomfort is felt.

Wall Seated Hamstring Stretch: involves sitting on the floor with your legs extended up against a wall, and your hips close to the wall. Hold this position for 30-60 seconds while reaching for your toes. This exercise targets the hamstrings, helping to improve flexibility and reduce muscle tension in the legs. Care should be taken to stop if any pain or discomfort is felt, and medical advice sought if necessary.

Wall Figure Four Hip Stretch: lie on your back with your feet up against a wall and knees bent. Cross one ankle over the opposite knee and slide your foot down the wall until you feel a stretch in your hip. Use your hand to gently push your knee out from your body. Hold this position for 30-60 seconds before switching sides. This exercise targets the hip muscles, helping to improve flexibility, reduce muscle tension, and prevent injury in the hips and lower back.

4.2 Strengthening Exercises

Wall Abdominal Crunch: is an effective exercise that targets your abs. To perform this workout, start by lying on your back with your legs up against the wall, knees bent, and feet flat. Place your hands behind your head and clench your core muscles. Lift your shoulders off the ground while keeping your core tight, then slowly lower yourself back down. Repeat this motion for 10-12 reps.

This exercise is a great way to strengthen your core muscles, which can improve your overall posture, stability, and balance. By using the wall as support, you can reduce the strain on your lower back and focus solely on engaging your abdominal muscles. The Wall Abdominal Crunch can be a challenging exercise, but with consistent practice, you can gradually increase your strength and endurance.

Wall Bridge exercise: is performed by lying on your back with your feet resting against a wall and your knees bent. By engaging your glutes and hamstrings, you lift your hips towards the ceiling and hold for a few seconds before lowering yourself back down. This movement is repeated 10 to 12 times, which provides an effective workout that targets the glute and hamstring muscles.

The Wall Bridge exercise is a great way to build strength and tone these specific muscle groups without putting too much pressure on the knees and lower back. It also helps to improve flexibility and mobility in the hips and lower body. Incorporating this exercise into your regular fitness routine can lead to better posture, balance, and overall fitness.

In summary, the Wall Bridge is a simple but effective exercise that targets the glutes and hamstrings while promoting better mobility and flexibility in the lower body.

The exercise named **"Wall Superman"** is designed to strengthen your back muscles. To perform this exercise, you need to lie down on your stomach with your hands on the floor and your feet pressed against a wall. Then, contract your back muscles and simultaneously lift your arms, chest, and knees off the ground. Hold this position for a few seconds before lowering yourself back down to the starting position. Repeat this movement for 10 to 12 times to complete one set.

This exercise is an effective way to target your back muscles, especially your lower back. By lifting your limbs and torso off the ground, you engage the muscles that support your spine, helping to improve your posture and prevent lower back pain. The movement also strengthens your upper back and shoulders, making it a great addition to any workout routine aimed at developing a stronger, healthier back.

Wall Leg Lifts: start by lying on your back with your legs stretched up against the wall. Slowly lower one leg towards the ground, keeping it straight, then lift it back up to the wall. Repeat this movement with the other leg and continue alternating for 10-12 repetitions.

This exercise is a great way to target the lower abs and hip flexors. By lifting and lowering your legs while they are against the wall, you engage these muscles in a controlled and effective way. Additionally, since your back is flat against the floor, there is minimal strain on your spine and neck.

Incorporating wall leg lifts into your workout routine can help to strengthen and tone your abs and hips. As with any exercise, be sure to use proper form and start with a manageable number of repetitions before increasing intensity.

Wall Knee Tucks exercise is a great way to target your abdominal muscles. To perform this exercise, start by lying on your back with your legs up against a wall. Your knees should be bent, and your feet should be flat against the wall. Engage your core muscles and bring your knees up towards your chest, keeping your feet flat against the wall. Hold this position for a moment before lowering your legs back down to the starting position. Repeat this movement for a total of 10-12 repetitions.

This exercise is an effective way to challenge your abs and improve their strength and endurance. The elevated leg position against the wall adds an extra level of resistance to the exercise, making it more challenging for your abdominal muscles. By incorporating the Wall Knee Tucks into your fitness routine, you can work towards achieving a stronger core and better overall fitness.

Wall Push-Ups with Alternating Leg Lifts: begin by standing in front of a wall and placing your hands at shoulder height on the wall. Perform a push-up, then raise one leg off the ground and hold it for several seconds before lowering it back down. Repeat the exercise with your other leg and continue alternating for 10-12 repetitions. This exercise is excellent for targeting several muscles, including your chest, shoulders, triceps, and abs. The push-up motion targets the upper body muscles, while the leg lift engages your core muscles. This exercise is particularly useful for people who are short on time or who do not have access to a gym. It can be done anywhere and requires no equipment, making it a convenient and effective addition to any workout routine.

Wall Side Leg Lifts: begin by standing parallel to a wall with one hand on it for balance. Ensure that both your hips and feet are facing forward. Now, lift your upper leg towards the wall, while keeping your balance and stability. Lower your leg back down and repeat the movement 10-12 times on each leg.

This exercise primarily targets the muscles on the outside of your thighs, specifically the abductor muscles. These muscles are responsible for stabilizing the pelvis and maintaining balance during movements such as walking, running, and jumping. Strengthening these muscles can help improve your overall lower body strength and stability, reducing the risk of injuries and improving athletic performance.

Wall Side Leg Lifts are an excellent exercise to add to your lower body workout routine. They can be performed anywhere with a wall for support and require no equipment, making them a convenient and effective exercise for building strong and toned thighs.

Wall Toe Taps exercise involves lying on your back with your legs extended up against a wall and tapping your toes against the wall for 10-12 repetitions, alternating between legs. This workout is primarily aimed at engaging and strengthening the abdominal muscles and hip flexors.

By maintaining the legs at a 90-degree angle against the wall, the abdominal muscles are required to work harder to stabilize the pelvis and prevent the lower back from arching. Meanwhile, the hip flexors are activated as they work to lift the legs off the ground and bring them towards the wall.

The Wall Toe Taps exercise is a low-impact workout that can be beneficial for individuals who are recovering from injuries or who have limited mobility. This exercise can be modified to suit different fitness levels by increasing or decreasing the number of repetitions or by adding ankle weights for added resistance.

Wall Bicycle Crunches, start by lying on your back with your legs extended up the wall, knees bent, and feet flat against the wall. Then, engage your abdominal muscles and twist your torso as you bring one elbow towards the opposite knee. Repeat this movement on the other side, alternating for 10-12 repetitions.

This exercise is an effective way to target your abdominal and oblique muscles. By lifting your legs up the wall, you create a stable base for your back, reducing the risk of strain or injury. The twisting motion of the exercise helps to engage your obliques and challenge your core stability. Additionally, the wall bicycle crunch can be modified by adjusting the speed and range of motion to suit your fitness level. Overall, incorporating wall bicycle crunches into your workout routine is a great way to strengthen your core and improve your overall fitness.

Wall Push-Ups With Hands On A Wall, begin by standing facing the wall with your hands positioned on the wall at shoulder height. Ensure that your body is straight and your chest, shoulders, and triceps are engaged. Execute the push-up by bending your elbows and leaning towards the wall, then return to the starting position. Repeat this process 10 to 12 times. This exercise is particularly useful for strengthening the chest, shoulders, and triceps muscles. By adjusting the distance between your feet and the wall, you can modify the intensity of the workout. Additionally, wall push-ups are an excellent choice for individuals who are new to fitness or have limited upper body strength, as they offer a low-impact way to build muscle and improve overall fitness. By incorporating wall push-ups into your exercise routine, you can develop strength, tone, and endurance in the upper body.

Wall Leg Lifts With A Resistance Band, lie on your side with your bottom leg resting against the wall. Wrap a resistance band around your top ankle and lift your top leg towards the wall while keeping your hips forward. Lower your leg back down and repeat this process 10 to 12 times on each leg. This exercise targets the muscles on the outside of your thighs, known as the abductors. Strengthening these muscles can improve your stability, balance, and overall lower body strength. The resistance band adds an extra challenge, helping to increase the intensity of the exercise and promote muscle growth. By regularly including wall leg lifts with a resistance band in your fitness routine, you can enhance your leg strength and improve your overall physical fitness.

Wall Single Leg Squats, begin by standing facing the wall with one hand on the wall for balance. Lift one leg off the ground and bend the other knee to perform a squat. Ensure that your knee does not go beyond your toes and that your back remains straight. Return to the starting position and repeat the exercise 10 to 12 times on each leg. This exercise primarily targets the quadriceps, hamstrings, and glutes muscles, which are essential for lower body strength and overall stability. The added balance challenge from performing the squats on one leg also engages your core muscles, providing an excellent full-body workout. Incorporating wall single leg squats into your exercise routine can help improve your balance, stability, and lower body strength, making it easier to perform daily activities and sports-related movements. By starting with a few repetitions and gradually increasing the number of repetitions, you can gradually build up your leg strength and endurance over time.

4.3 Sculpting Exercises

Wall Plank Exercise, place your hands on the wall at shoulder height and move your feet back until your body forms a straight line from your head to your heels. Engage your core muscles by pulling your belly button towards your spine and holding this position for 30 to 60 seconds. The wall plank is an effective exercise that targets your core, arms, and shoulders. By holding your body in a straight line, you are engaging your abdominal muscles and lower back muscles, which help to improve your overall posture and core strength. Additionally, the wall plank strengthens your arms and shoulders as you hold yourself up against the wall. As you become stronger, you can increase the amount of time you hold the position, or you can try performing the exercise with your feet elevated on a bench or stability ball. Incorporating the wall plank into your fitness routine can help you build a strong core and upper body, improve your posture, and reduce the risk of injury during other exercises or daily activities.

Wall Push-Up exercise involves standing facing the wall and placing your hands on the wall at shoulder height. Step back with your feet until your body forms a straight line from your head to your heels. Bend your elbows and lower your body towards the wall, then push back up to the starting position. Repeat this process 10 to 12 times. This exercise primarily targets the chest, shoulders, and triceps muscles, which are essential for upper body strength and stability. By adjusting the distance between your feet and the wall, you can modify the intensity of the workout. The wall push-up is an excellent choice for individuals who are new to fitness or have limited upper body strength, as it provides a low-impact way to build muscle and improve overall fitness. By regularly incorporating wall push-ups into your exercise routine, you can develop strength, tone, and endurance in the upper body, making it easier to perform daily activities and other exercises.

Wall Sit exercise, start by standing with your back against the wall. Slide down the wall until your thighs are parallel to the floor, forming a 90-degree angle at your knees. Hold this position for 30 to 60 seconds before returning to the starting position. This exercise targets the quadriceps and glutes muscles, which are essential for lower body strength and overall stability. The wall sit is a great exercise for developing isometric strength, which is the ability to hold a static position for an extended period. Additionally, this exercise can help improve your posture and increase your endurance. By regularly incorporating wall sits into your fitness routine, you can build strength and endurance in your lower body, making it easier to perform daily activities and other exercises. You can increase the intensity of the workout by holding a weight or a medicine ball in front of you while performing the wall sit.

Wall Squat is an exercise that targets the quadriceps and glutes while also engaging the core muscles. To perform this exercise, stand facing a wall with your feet hip-width apart and your hands resting on the wall. Slowly slide down the wall while maintaining a straight back and engaging your core until your thighs are parallel to the floor. Hold this position for 10 to 15 seconds, then gradually return to the starting position. You can repeat this exercise 10 to 12 times more for an effective workout. By performing this exercise regularly, you can strengthen your lower body muscles, improve your posture, and increase your overall physical fitness. It is essential to maintain proper form throughout the exercise to avoid any injuries or strains.

Wall Tricep Dips are an effective exercise that target the triceps. To perform this exercise, start by sitting on the floor with your back against the wall and your legs extended in front of you. Place your hands on the wall behind you, shoulder-width apart. Then, bend your elbows to lower your body towards the floor, and pause briefly before returning to the starting position. Repeat this movement for 10-12 reps.

The wall tricep dips can be a challenging exercise, as it requires significant upper body strength to lift and lower your body weight. However, it is a great exercise to tone and strengthen the triceps, which are the muscles located on the back of your upper arms. This exercise is ideal for anyone looking to improve their arm strength, especially those who may not have access to equipment like dumbbells or resistance bands.

Wall Leg Press exercise, start by standing facing a wall with your hands placed on the wall at shoulder height. Lift one leg off the floor and place the foot against the wall. Slowly lower your body by bending the standing leg, keeping your back straight, until the thigh of the lifted leg is parallel to the ground. Push back up to the starting position and repeat the movement for 10-12 repetitions before switching to the other leg.

The Wall Leg Press primarily targets the quadriceps and glutes muscles, making it an effective lower body workout. This exercise requires no equipment, making it an excellent choice for those who prefer to exercise at home or have limited equipment available. It can also be a good option for individuals with knee pain as it places less stress on the knee joint than traditional squats or lunges. Overall, incorporating the Wall Leg Press into your fitness routine can help to improve lower body strength and endurance.

Wall Lunge is a lower body exercise that targets multiple muscle groups, including the quadriceps, glutes, and hamstrings. To perform this exercise, start by standing facing a wall and place your hands at shoulder height on the wall. Step back with one foot and lower your body into a lunge position, making sure your front knee is directly over your ankle. Push back up to the starting position and repeat the movement 10 to 12 times on each leg.

By engaging these muscle groups, the Wall Lunge can help improve your lower body strength and stability. Additionally, this exercise can be an effective way to improve your balance and coordination, making it a great addition to your regular workout routine.

Overall, the Wall Lunge is a simple yet effective exercise that can provide a challenging workout for your lower body. Incorporating it into your routine can help you build strength, improve your balance and coordination, and enhance your overall fitness level.

Wall Hip Bridge is a simple yet effective exercise that targets the glutes and lower back. To perform this exercise, lie on your back with your feet against a wall and your knees bent. Next, squeeze your glutes and lift your hips off the floor for 10 to 15 seconds. Then, lower your hips back to the floor and repeat the movement for 10 to 12 repetitions.

This exercise can help improve the strength and tone of your glutes and lower back, which can benefit your overall fitness level and help reduce the risk of injury. Additionally, the Wall Hip Bridge can be a great exercise for individuals who experience lower back pain, as it can help alleviate discomfort and improve spinal alignment.

Overall, the Wall Hip Bridge is a simple yet effective exercise that can provide a challenging workout for your glutes and lower back. By incorporating it into your regular fitness routine, you can help improve your strength, mobility, and overall health.

Wall Chest Press is a bodyweight exercise that targets the chest, shoulders, and triceps. To perform this exercise, stand facing away from a wall and place your hands at shoulder height on the wall. Next, bend your elbows and lower your body towards the wall, keeping your core engaged and your back straight. Finally, push back up to the starting position and repeat the movement for 10 to 12 repetitions.

By engaging these muscle groups, the Wall Chest Press can help improve upper body strength and tone. Additionally, this exercise can be a great alternative to traditional chest press exercises that require equipment, making it a convenient option for those who prefer to workout at home or while traveling.

Overall, the Wall Chest Press is a simple yet effective exercise that can provide a challenging workout for your chest, shoulders, and triceps. Incorporating it into your regular fitness routine can help improve your upper body strength, tone, and overall health.

Wall Leg Circles is a lower body exercise that targets the glutes and hip flexors. To perform this exercise, stand facing a wall with your hands at shoulder height on the wall. Next, lift one leg off the floor and draw circles with your foot in the opposite direction. Repeat the movement for 10 to 12 repetitions on each leg.

By engaging these muscle groups, the Wall Leg Circles can help improve your lower body strength, balance, and stability. Additionally, this exercise can be an effective way to improve your flexibility and range of motion in the hips.

Overall, the Wall Leg Circles is a simple yet effective exercise that can provide a challenging workout for your lower body. By incorporating it into your regular fitness routine, you can help improve your lower body strength, balance, flexibility, and overall health.

Wall Inner Thigh Squeeze is an exercise that targets the muscles in the inner thighs. To perform this exercise, stand facing a wall with your feet hip-width apart and your hands on the wall. Next, squeeze a small ball or pillow between your knees as you lower into a wall squat. Hold the position for around 10 to 15 seconds, then release and return to the starting position. Repeat the movement for 10 to 12 repetitions.

By engaging the muscles in the inner thighs, the Wall Inner Thigh Squeeze can help improve your lower body strength and tone. Additionally, this exercise can be a great way to target specific areas of the body and can be easily modified by using a different-sized ball or adjusting the duration of the hold.

Overall, the Wall Inner Thigh Squeeze is a simple yet effective exercise that can provide a challenging workout for your inner thighs. By incorporating it into your regular fitness routine, you can help improve your lower body strength, tone, and overall health.

Wall Single Leg Deadlift is a lower body exercise that targets the hamstrings, glutes, and lower back. To perform this exercise, stand facing a wall with your hands at shoulder height on the wall. Next, hinge forward at the hips and extend your elevated leg behind you as you lower your body towards the wall. Keep your core engaged and your back straight throughout the movement. Finally, return to the starting position and repeat the exercise for 10 to 12 repetitions on each leg.

By engaging these muscle groups, the Wall Single Leg Deadlift can help improve your lower body strength, balance, and stability. Additionally, this exercise can be an effective way to improve your posture and reduce the risk of lower back pain.

Overall, the Wall Single Leg Deadlift is a challenging exercise that can provide a great workout for your hamstrings, glutes, and lower back. By incorporating it into your regular fitness routine, you can help improve your lower body strength, balance, and overall health.

Wall Pike is a challenging exercise that targets the shoulders, abs, and hamstrings. To perform this exercise, start in a plank position with your feet against a wall and your hands on the ground. Next, lift your hips towards the sky and walk your feet up the wall towards your hands, keeping your legs straight. Hold the position for a few seconds before lowering back down and repeating the movement for 10 to 12 repetitions.

By engaging these muscle groups, the Wall Pike can help improve your upper body and core strength, as well as your flexibility and mobility. Additionally, this exercise can be a great way to challenge yourself and add variety to your workout routine.

Overall, the Wall Pike is a challenging exercise that can provide a great workout for your shoulders, abs, and hamstrings. By incorporating it into your regular fitness routine, you can help improve your upper body and core strength, flexibility, and overall health.

Wall Scissor Kicks is an exercise that targets the abs and hip flexors. To perform this exercise, lie on your back with your legs up against a wall, making sure that your heels are in contact with the wall and your toes are pointing up. Next, scissor your legs up and down for 10 to 12 repetitions, alternating which leg is on top.

By engaging these muscle groups, the Wall Scissor Kicks can help improve your core strength and flexibility, as well as your balance and stability. Additionally, this exercise can be a great way to target specific areas of the body and can be easily modified to increase or decrease the intensity.

Overall, the Wall Scissor Kicks is a simple yet effective exercise that can provide a great workout for your abs and hip flexors. By incorporating it into your regular fitness routine, you can help improve your core strength, flexibility, and overall health.

Wall Roll-Up is an exercise that targets the abs and spine. To perform this exercise, sit on the floor with your back against a wall and your legs extended in front of you. Next, roll your spine up the wall with your arms reaching towards your toes. Slowly lower yourself back down and repeat the movement for 10 to 12 repetitions.

By engaging these muscle groups, the Wall Roll-Up can help improve your core strength and spinal mobility, as well as your posture and overall fitness level. Additionally, this exercise can be a great way to relieve tension and discomfort in the back and neck.

Overall, the Wall Roll-Up is a simple yet effective exercise that can provide a great workout for your abs and spine. By incorporating it into your regular fitness routine, you can help improve your core strength, spinal mobility, and overall health.

Wall Side Plank is an exercise that targets the oblique muscles and shoulders. To perform this exercise, start in a plank position with your feet against a wall and one hand on the ground. Next, rotate your bottom foot to the outside and elevate your other hand towards the ceiling, holding the position for a few seconds before lowering back down. Repeat the movement on the opposite side and alternate for 10 to 12 repetitions.

By engaging these muscle groups, the Wall Side Plank can help improve your core strength, stability, and balance, as well as your shoulder mobility and strength. Additionally, this exercise can be a great way to target specific areas of the body and can be easily modified to increase or decrease the intensity.

Overall, the Wall Side Plank is a challenging exercise that can provide a great workout for your oblique muscles and shoulders. By incorporating it into your regular fitness routine, you can help improve your core strength, stability, and overall health.

Wall Tucks is an exercise that targets the abs. To perform this exercise, start in a plank position with your feet against a wall and your hands on the ground. Next, round your spine and contract your abs as you bring your knees to your chest. Extend your legs back to the plank position and repeat the movement for 10 to 12 repetitions.

By engaging these muscle groups, the Wall Tucks can help improve your core strength, stability, and balance. Additionally, this exercise can be a great way to challenge yourself and add variety to your workout routine.

Overall, the Wall Tucks is a simple yet effective exercise that can provide a great workout for your abs. By incorporating it into your regular fitness routine, you can help improve your core strength, stability, and overall health.

Wall Climbers is an exercise that targets the abs and hip flexors. To perform this exercise, start in a plank position with your feet against a wall and your hands on the ground. Next, bring one knee in towards your chest, then stretch it back out and bring the other knee in. Alternate between the two knees for a total of 10 to 12 repetitions.

By engaging these muscle groups, the Wall Climbers can help improve your core strength, stability, and balance, as well as your hip flexibility and mobility. Additionally, this exercise can be a great way to add variety to your workout routine and challenge yourself.

Overall, the Wall Climbers is a simple yet effective exercise that can provide a great workout for your abs and hip flexors. By incorporating it into your regular fitness routine, you can help improve your core strength, stability, flexibility, and overall health.

Wall Scapular Slide is an exercise that targets the muscles in the upper back. To perform this exercise, stand facing a wall with your arms at shoulder height and your palms against the wall. Next, move your shoulder blades down towards your hips, then back up towards your ears. Repeat the movement for 10 to 12 repetitions.

By engaging these muscle groups, the Wall Scapular Slide can help improve your posture, reduce tension and discomfort in the upper back, and improve your overall upper body strength and stability.

Overall, the Wall Scapular Slide is a simple yet effective exercise that can provide a great workout for your upper back. By incorporating it into your regular fitness routine, you can help improve your posture, reduce discomfort and tension in the upper back, and improve your overall upper body strength and stability.

Wall Knee Folds is an exercise that targets the abs and hip flexors. To perform this exercise, lie on your back with your legs up against a wall, your knees bent, and your feet flat against the wall. Next, bring your knees towards your chest and hold the position for a few seconds before stretching your legs out again. Repeat the movement for 10 to 12 repetitions.

By engaging these muscle groups, the Wall Knee Folds can help improve your core strength and stability, as well as your hip flexibility and mobility. Additionally, this exercise can be a great way to relieve tension and discomfort in the lower back and hips.

Overall, the Wall Knee Folds is a simple yet effective exercise that can provide a great workout for your abs and hip flexors. By incorporating it into your regular fitness routine, you can help improve your core strength, flexibility, and overall health.

Wall Spiderman Climb is an exercise that targets the abdominals, oblique muscles, and hip flexors. To perform this exercise, start in a plank position with your feet against a wall and your hands on the ground. Next, bring one knee up to your elbow, then extend it and bring the second knee up to your opposite elbow. Alternate between the two knees for a total of 10 to 12 repetitions.

By engaging these muscle groups, the Wall Spiderman Climb can help improve your core strength, stability, and balance, as well as your hip flexibility and mobility. Additionally, this exercise can be a great way to challenge yourself and add variety to your workout routine.

Overall, the Wall Spiderman Climb is a challenging exercise that can provide a great workout for your abs, oblique muscles, and hip flexors. By incorporating it into your regular fitness routine, you can help improve your core strength, stability, flexibility, and overall health.

Wall Plank with Leg Lifts is an exercise that targets the glutes and abs. To perform this exercise, start in a plank position with your feet against a wall and your hands on the ground. Next, lift one leg towards the ceiling, keeping it straight and your glutes engaged. Lower yourself back down and repeat the movement on the opposite leg for 10 to 12 repetitions.

By engaging these muscle groups, the Wall Plank with Leg Lifts can help improve your core strength, stability, and balance, as well as your gluteal muscle strength and definition. Additionally, this exercise can be a great way to challenge yourself and add variety to your workout routine.

Overall, the Wall Plank with Leg Lifts is a challenging exercise that can provide a great workout for your glutes and abs. By incorporating it into your regular fitness routine, you can help improve your core strength, stability, flexibility, and overall health.

Wall Lateral Leg Swings is an exercise that targets the muscles on the outside of the thighs. To perform this exercise, stand facing a wall with your hands on the wall for balance. Next, swing one leg to the side and then back in towards the wall. Repeat the movement for 10 to 12 repetitions on the opposite leg.

By engaging these muscle groups, the Wall Lateral Leg Swings can help improve your hip mobility and stability, as well as tone and define the muscles on the outside of the thighs. Additionally, this exercise can be a great way to add variety to your workout routine and improve your overall lower body strength.

Overall, the Wall Lateral Leg Swings is a simple yet effective exercise that can provide a great workout for the muscles on the outside of your thighs. By incorporating it into your regular fitness routine, you can help improve your hip mobility, tone and define your lower body muscles, and improve your overall health.

Wall Side Plank with Leg Lifts is an exercise that targets the glutes and outer thighs. To perform this exercise, start in a side plank position with your feet against a wall and one hand on the ground. Next, lift your upper leg towards the ceiling, keeping it straight and your glutes engaged. Lower yourself back down and repeat the movement for 10 to 12 repetitions.

By engaging these muscle groups, the Wall Side Plank with Leg Lifts can help improve your core strength, stability, and balance, as well as tone and define the muscles in your glutes and outer thighs. Additionally, this exercise can be a great way to challenge yourself and add variety to your workout routine.

Overall, the Wall Side Plank with Leg Lifts is a challenging exercise that can provide a great workout for your glutes and outer thighs. By incorporating it into your regular fitness routine, you can help improve your core strength, stability, flexibility, and overall health.

CHAPTER 5: WALL PILATES 30-DAY PROGRAMS

After learning about wall Pilates and the various exercises that can help you tone and reshape your body, it's time to put your knowledge into action. In this chapter, we'll provide you with a 30-day program to help you achieve your fitness goals.

It's important to note that consistency is key when it comes to any fitness program. For the best results, it's recommended that you perform these exercises at least 4-5 times a week. Additionally, it's crucial to listen to your body and modify any exercises that feel uncomfortable or painful. Pushing through pain can lead to injury and setbacks, so it's essential to prioritize safety and well-being.

There are different plans provided, so you can choose the one that best suits your needs and goals. Alternatively, you can mix and match different plans to create a personalized workout routine that works best for you. It's important to find a balance between challenging yourself and not pushing your body beyond its limits. If you're new to physical activity or have been inactive for a while, it's advisable to gradually increase the intensity of your workouts to avoid injury and promote a positive experience. Having a positive and enjoyable workout experience is essential for success.

Each plan comes with a recommended number of repetitions to be effective and bring visible results. However, it's important to note that these recommendations are not one-size-fits-all. Depending on your level of fitness and your specific goals, you may need to adjust the number of repetitions and frequency of workouts to suit your needs. It's essential to personalize your workout routine to ensure that you're challenging yourself appropriately while also avoiding injury and burnout.

One of the benefits of wall Pilates is that it can be easily adapted to accommodate different fitness levels and goals. For example, if your goal is to increase muscle tone and definition, you may want to focus on exercises that target specific muscle groups, such as the legs or arms. On the other hand, if your goal is to improve overall flexibility and balance, you may want to focus on exercises that target the core and incorporate full-body movements.

Ultimately, the key to success with any fitness program is to stay committed and consistent. It's essential to make exercise a regular part of your routine and prioritize your health and well-being. With the help of this 30-day program and your own dedication, you can achieve your fitness goals and feel stronger, healthier, and more confident in your body.

5.1 Posture and Core Routine Exercises (10/15 Minutes)

This routine is designed to improve your posture and strengthen your core muscles, including your abs and back muscles. By improving your posture, you'll look taller and more confident, and your body will function more efficiently. A strong core is also essential for maintaining a healthy spine and preventing back pain. This type of plan is very useful for those who are approaching physical activity after some time of inactivity or for those who do sedentary work and need to wake up their muscles without trauma. It is also the basic activity for those approaching wall Pilates exercises for the first time and is preparatory to more complex exercises. It is essential that these exercises are done correctly, maintaining proper posture, breathing and timing.

In this plan, we've included a selection of exercises that will be thoroughly explained in the following pages. As you progress and become more comfortable with the workouts, feel free to incorporate additional exercises to challenge yourself further.

WALL POSTURE CHECK (EXERCISE A)

Stand with your back against the wall and your feet hip-width apart. Check your posture and make sure your shoulders are back, your chest is lifted, and your chin is parallel to the ground. Hold the position for 30 seconds. Extend your arms, at shoulder height, and hold this position for 60 seconds.

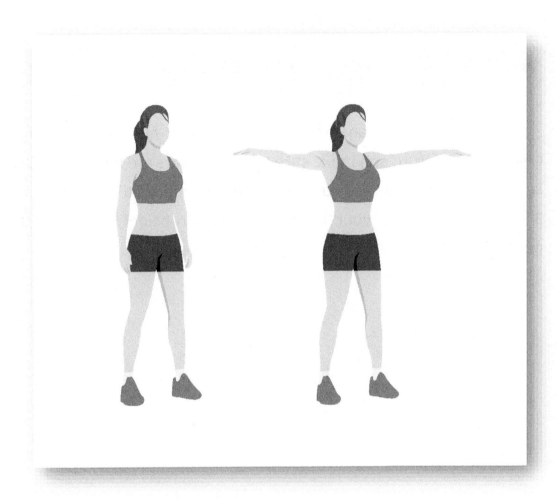

WALL PLANK   (EXERCISE B)

Start in a plank position with feet against the wall and hands on the floor. The whole body should be aligned. Keep the core engaged and hold the position for 30-60 seconds. The position should be held without excessive effort otherwise you can hold the same position but with your arms bent i.e. with the weight on your elbows. Once trained you will be able to perform the position with arms extended and hands on the ground. (see page 36)

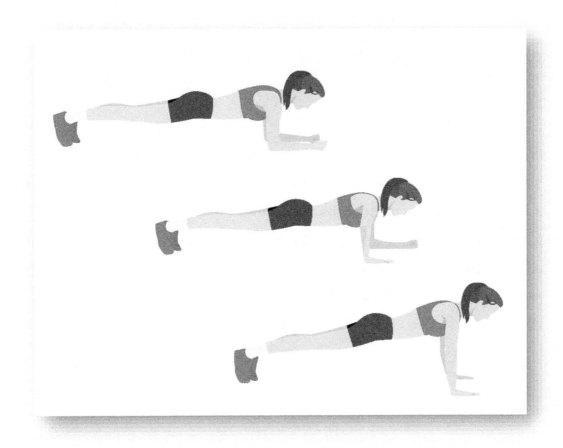

WALL CAT-COW STRETCH   (EXERCISE C)

Start on your hands and knees with your hands against the wall. Arch your back toward the ceiling, then round your spine toward the wall. Repeat for 10-12 repetitions and combine breathing. Inhale as you arch toward the ceiling and exhale as you stretch toward the wall.

* Please note that your hands should be resting on the wall and your arms outstretched.

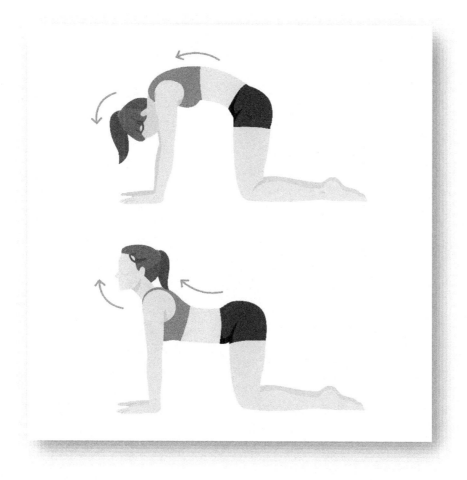

WALL HAMSTRING STRETCH   (EXERCISE D)

Lie on your back with your legs stretched up against a wall and your hips near the wall. Flex your feet and gently bring your toes closer to your shins to deepen the stretch. Hold this position for 30 to 60 seconds. 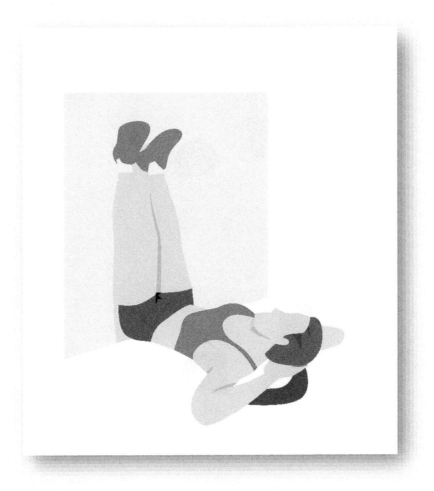(see page 26)

WALL ABDOMINAL CRUNCH   (EXERCISE E)

Lie on your back with your legs against the wall and your hands behind your head. Bring your torso closer to your knees, engaging your abs. Lower yourself down and repeat for 10 to 12 repetitions. The movement does not need to be large and should come mainly from contracting the abdominals. (see page 29)

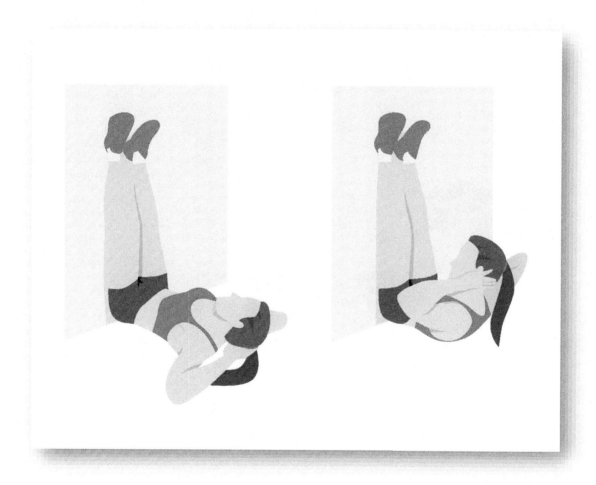

WALL SUPERMAN   (EXERCISE F)

Lie on your stomach with your hands on the floor and your feet against the wall. Lift your arms, chest, and legs off the ground, contracting your back muscles. Lower back down and repeat for 10-15 repetitions. This exercise aims to strengthen the back muscles to benefit posture. (see page 30)

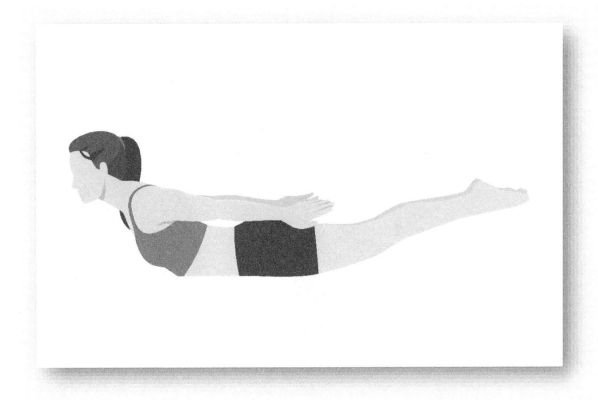

30-DAY Posture Routine CHART

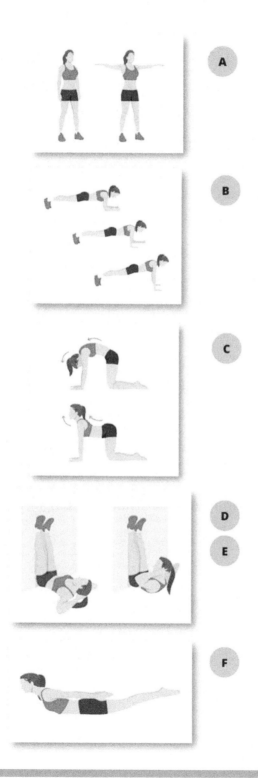

A

B

C

D

E

F

WEEK 1 (1-6 DAYS)

A/B: 10 OF EACH X 2 REPS

C/D: 10 OF EACH X 2 REPS

E/F: 10 OF EACH X 2 REPS

DAY 6: REST

WEEK 2 (7-12 DAYS)

A/B: 10 OF EACH X 2 REPS

C/D: 12 OF EACH X 2 REPS

E/F: 12 OF EACH X 2 REPS

DAY 12: REST

WEEK 3 (13-18 DAYS)

A/B: 10 OF EACH X 2 REPS

C/D: 12 OF EACH X 2 REPS

E/F: 12 OF EACH X 2 REPS

DAY 18: REST

WEEK 4   (19-24 DAYS)

A/B: 12 OF EACH X 2 REPS

C/D: 15 OF EACH X 2 REPS

E/F: 15 OF EACH X 2 REPS

DAY 24: REST

WEEK 5   (25-30 DAYS)

A/B: 12 OF EACH X 2 REPS

C/D: 15 OF EACH X 2 REPS

E/F: 15 OF EACH X 2 REPS

DAY 30: REST

This exercise routine has been created with the aim of enhancing your coordination, stability, and balance, which can reduce the risk of falls. Through better balance, you will also be able to carry out other exercises with more precision and control.

Falls are a major concern, particularly in older adults. By incorporating exercises that specifically target balance and stability, it is possible to lower the chances of falls and the associated injuries. Improving balance and stability can also benefit people in their daily lives, such as being able to walk or stand for longer periods without feeling unsteady.

Furthermore, mastering balance and stability can have a positive effect on other areas of your fitness routine. It can enable you to perform exercises that require more coordination and focus, such as yoga or weightlifting, with greater ease and precision. Overall, focusing on improving your balance and stability is a smart investment in your fitness and overall health.

WALL SQUAT HOLD   (EXERCISE G)

Stand with your back against the wall and your feet hip-width apart.
Lower into a squat position and hold the position for 30-60 seconds.
(see page 38)

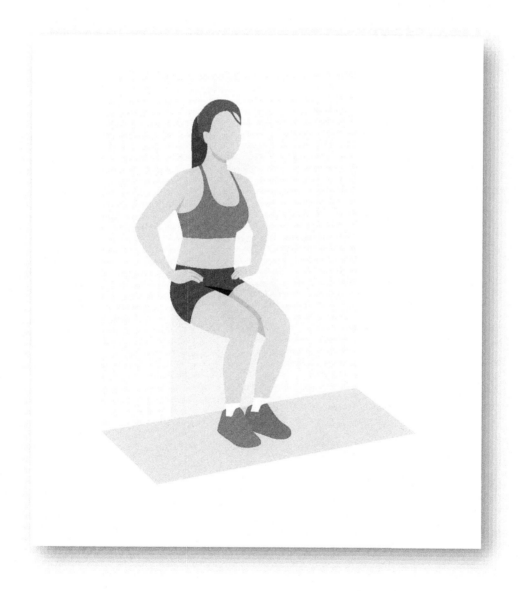

WALL SIT   (EXERCISE H)

Stand with your back against the wall. Slide along the wall until your thighs are parallel to the floor, forming a 90-degree angle at the knees. Extend one leg. Hold this position for 30 to 60 seconds before returning to the starting position. Alternate with the other leg and repeat. (see page 38)

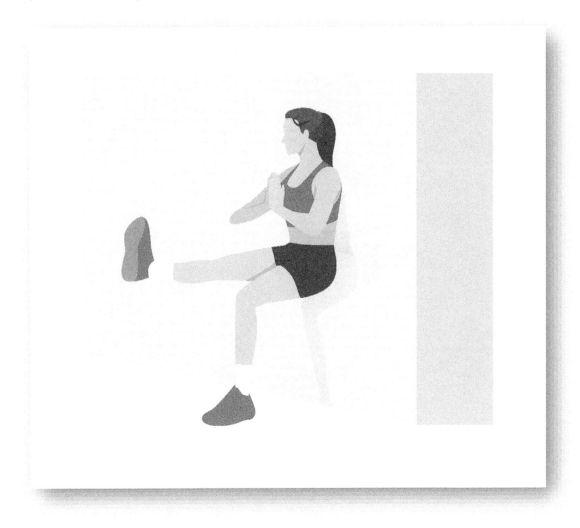

WALL LEG SWINGS   (EXERCISE I)

Stand sideways to the wall and rest one hand on the wall for balance. Swing one leg, opposite the resting hand, forward and backward while keeping the muscle active. Then switch legs. Repeat for 10 to 12 repetitions. (see page 51)

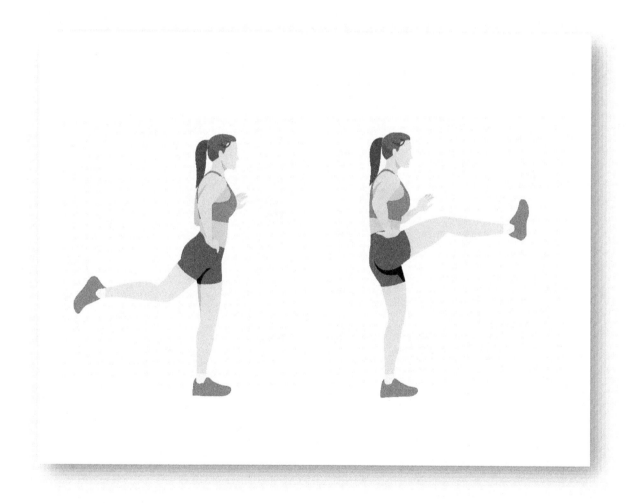

WALL LEG CIRCLES   (EXERCISE J)

Stand facing a wall with your hands at shoulder height on the wall. Next, lift one leg off the floor and draw circles with your foot in the opposite direction. Repeat the movement for 10 to 12 repetitions on each leg.(see page 42)

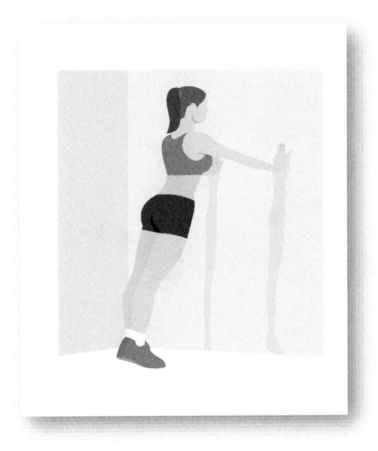

WALL SIDE KEG SWINGS   (EXERCISE K)

Stand sideways to the wall and rest one hand on the wall for balance. Swing one leg, opposite the supported hand, toward the wall and outward while keeping the muscle active and in control of the leg. Then switch legs. Repeat for 10 to 12 repetitions.

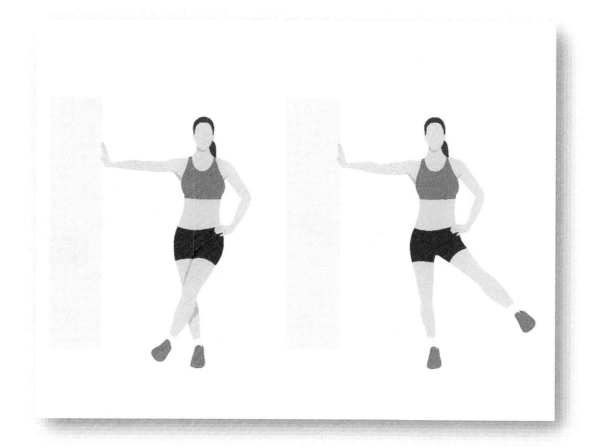

WALL KNEE TUCKS (EXERCISE L)

Lie on your back with your feet against the wall and knees bent. Engage your core muscles and bring your knees toward your chest. Hold this position for a moment before lowering your legs back to the starting position. Repeat this movement for a total of 10-12 repetitions. (see page 31)

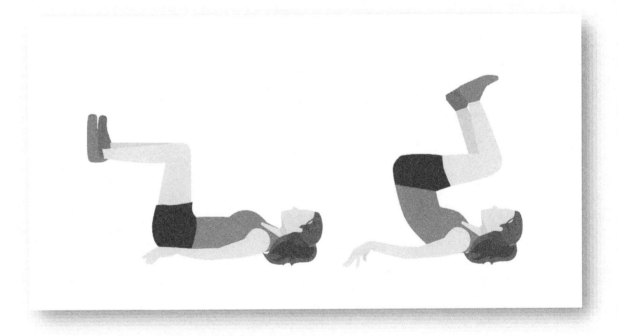

WALL BICYCLE CRUNCHES   (EXERCISE M)

Lie on your back with your hands behind your head, legs bent and feet against the wall. Bring one elbow toward the opposite knee, then switch sides. Repeat for 10 to 12 repetitions. (see page 34)

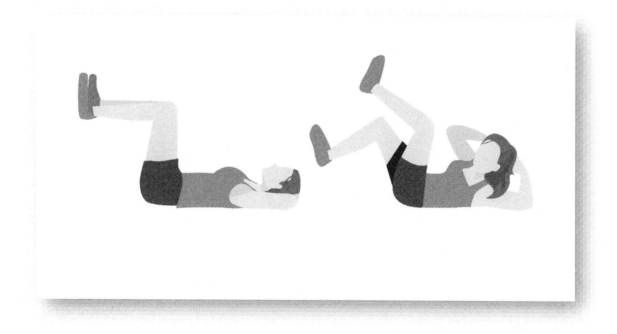

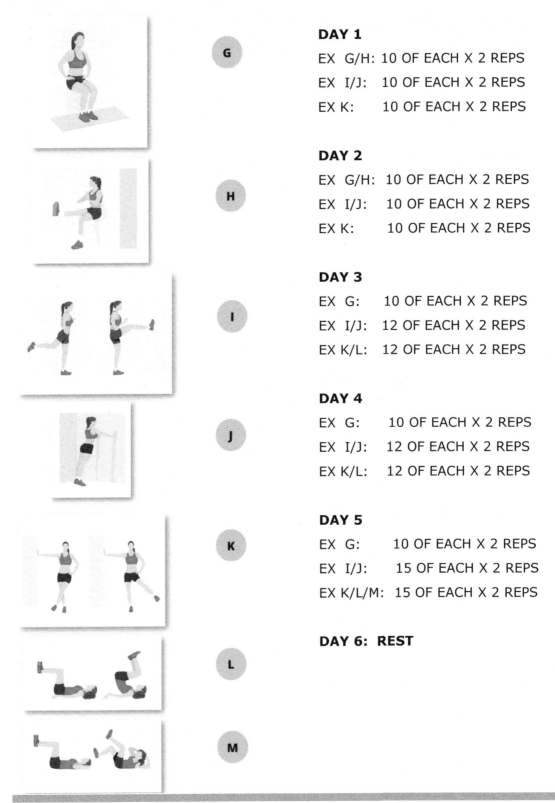

DAY 1

EX G/H: 10 OF EACH X 2 REPS

EX I/J: 10 OF EACH X 2 REPS

EX K: 10 OF EACH X 2 REPS

DAY 2

EX G/H: 10 OF EACH X 2 REPS

EX I/J: 10 OF EACH X 2 REPS

EX K: 10 OF EACH X 2 REPS

DAY 3

EX G: 10 OF EACH X 2 REPS

EX I/J: 12 OF EACH X 2 REPS

EX K/L: 12 OF EACH X 2 REPS

DAY 4

EX G: 10 OF EACH X 2 REPS

EX I/J: 12 OF EACH X 2 REPS

EX K/L: 12 OF EACH X 2 REPS

DAY 5

EX G: 10 OF EACH X 2 REPS

EX I/J: 15 OF EACH X 2 REPS

EX K/L/M: 15 OF EACH X 2 REPS

DAY 6: REST

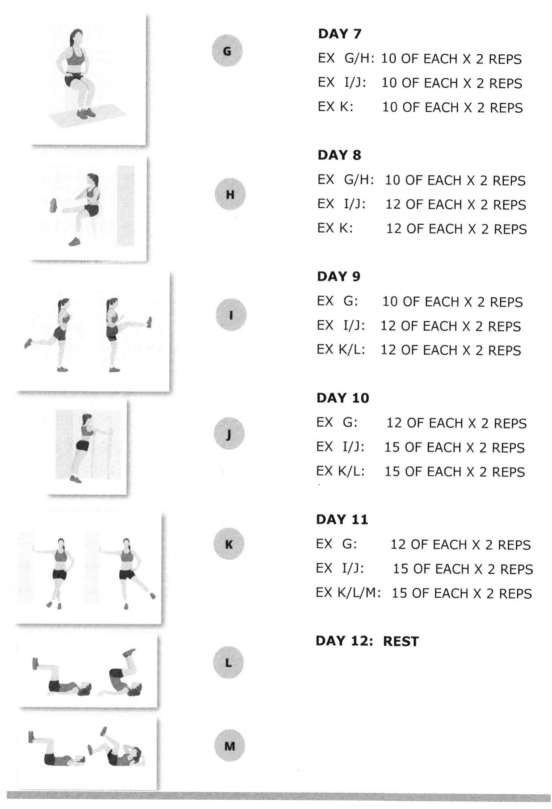

DAY 7

EX G/H: 10 OF EACH X 2 REPS

EX I/J: 10 OF EACH X 2 REPS

EX K: 10 OF EACH X 2 REPS

DAY 8

EX G/H: 10 OF EACH X 2 REPS

EX I/J: 12 OF EACH X 2 REPS

EX K: 12 OF EACH X 2 REPS

DAY 9

EX G: 10 OF EACH X 2 REPS

EX I/J: 12 OF EACH X 2 REPS

EX K/L: 12 OF EACH X 2 REPS

DAY 10

EX G: 12 OF EACH X 2 REPS

EX I/J: 15 OF EACH X 2 REPS

EX K/L: 15 OF EACH X 2 REPS

DAY 11

EX G: 12 OF EACH X 2 REPS

EX I/J: 15 OF EACH X 2 REPS

EX K/L/M: 15 OF EACH X 2 REPS

DAY 12: REST

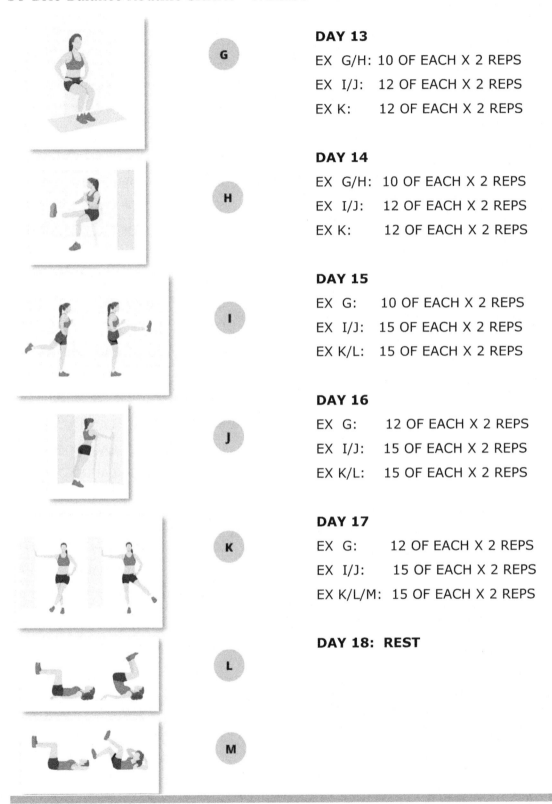

DAY 13

EX G/H: 10 OF EACH X 2 REPS

EX I/J: 12 OF EACH X 2 REPS

EX K: 12 OF EACH X 2 REPS

DAY 14

EX G/H: 10 OF EACH X 2 REPS

EX I/J: 12 OF EACH X 2 REPS

EX K: 12 OF EACH X 2 REPS

DAY 15

EX G: 10 OF EACH X 2 REPS

EX I/J: 15 OF EACH X 2 REPS

EX K/L: 15 OF EACH X 2 REPS

DAY 16

EX G: 12 OF EACH X 2 REPS

EX I/J: 15 OF EACH X 2 REPS

EX K/L: 15 OF EACH X 2 REPS

DAY 17

EX G: 12 OF EACH X 2 REPS

EX I/J: 15 OF EACH X 2 REPS

EX K/L/M: 15 OF EACH X 2 REPS

DAY 18: REST

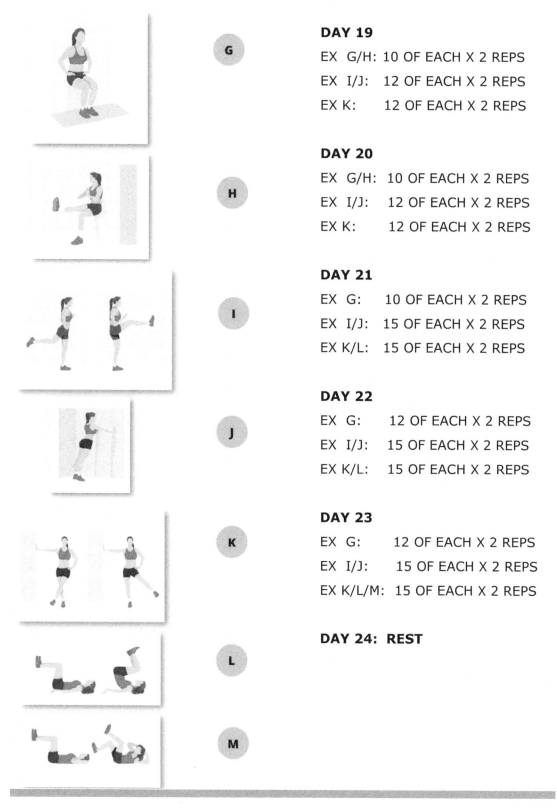

DAY 19

EX G/H: 10 OF EACH X 2 REPS

EX I/J: 12 OF EACH X 2 REPS

EX K: 12 OF EACH X 2 REPS

DAY 20

EX G/H: 10 OF EACH X 2 REPS

EX I/J: 12 OF EACH X 2 REPS

EX K: 12 OF EACH X 2 REPS

DAY 21

EX G: 10 OF EACH X 2 REPS

EX I/J: 15 OF EACH X 2 REPS

EX K/L: 15 OF EACH X 2 REPS

DAY 22

EX G: 12 OF EACH X 2 REPS

EX I/J: 15 OF EACH X 2 REPS

EX K/L: 15 OF EACH X 2 REPS

DAY 23

EX G: 12 OF EACH X 2 REPS

EX I/J: 15 OF EACH X 2 REPS

EX K/L/M: 15 OF EACH X 2 REPS

DAY 24: REST

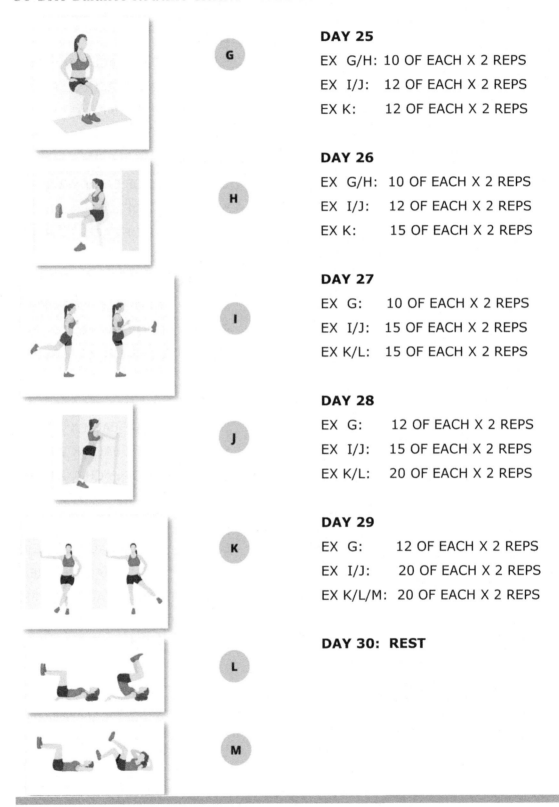

DAY 25

EX G/H: 10 OF EACH X 2 REPS

EX I/J: 12 OF EACH X 2 REPS

EX K: 12 OF EACH X 2 REPS

DAY 26

EX G/H: 10 OF EACH X 2 REPS

EX I/J: 12 OF EACH X 2 REPS

EX K: 15 OF EACH X 2 REPS

DAY 27

EX G: 10 OF EACH X 2 REPS

EX I/J: 15 OF EACH X 2 REPS

EX K/L: 15 OF EACH X 2 REPS

DAY 28

EX G: 12 OF EACH X 2 REPS

EX I/J: 15 OF EACH X 2 REPS

EX K/L: 20 OF EACH X 2 REPS

DAY 29

EX G: 12 OF EACH X 2 REPS

EX I/J: 20 OF EACH X 2 REPS

EX K/L/M: 20 OF EACH X 2 REPS

DAY 30: REST

This workout plan aims to enhance your abdominal strength and increase your flexibility. The benefits of improving your flexibility include increased mobility and reduced pain. With better flexibility, your body can move more easily and naturally. Additionally, a stronger core helps maintain good posture and provides support for your spine.

By practicing this routine regularly, you can expect to notice improvements in both areas. The exercises are designed to challenge and engage your abdominal muscles while also stretching and lengthening other muscles in your body. As you progress, you may find that you're able to move with more ease and less discomfort in your daily life.

It's important to remember that flexibility and strength take time to develop, so be patient with yourself and stay committed to the routine. With consistency and dedication, you can achieve the benefits of a stronger, more flexible body.

WALL SQUAT HOLD   (EXERCISE G)

Stand with your back against the wall and your feet hip-width apart.
Lower into a squat position and hold the position for 30-60 seconds.
(see page 38)

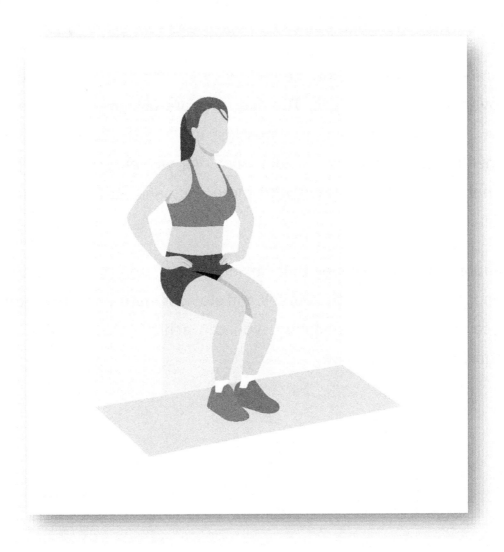

WALL CHEST STRETCH   (EXERCISE N)

Stand facing away from a wall and put one hand on it at shoulder height. Turn your body away from the wall until you feel a stretch in your chest. Hold this for 30-60 seconds before switching sides. (see page 26)

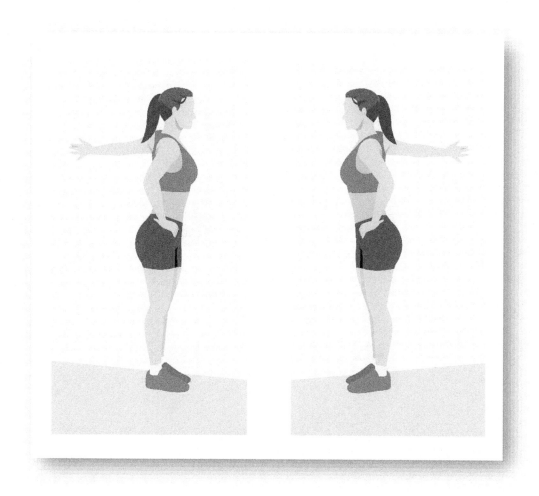

WALL LEG SWINGS   (EXERCISE I)

Stand sideways to the wall and rest one hand on the wall for balance. Swing one leg, opposite the resting hand, forward and backward while keeping the muscle active. Then switch legs. Repeat for 10 to 12 repetitions. (see page 51)

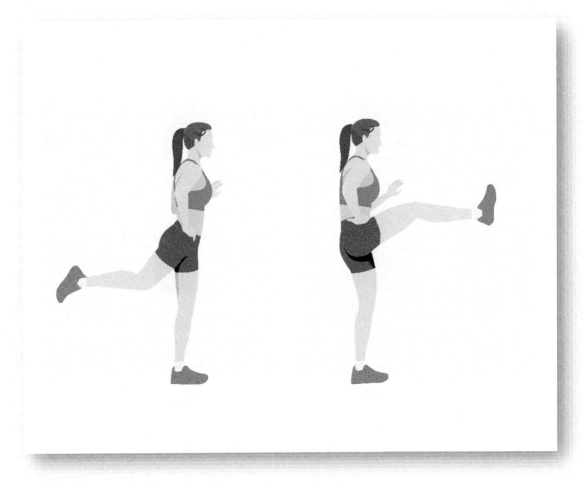

WALL PUSH-UPS WITH HANDS ON WALL (EXERCISE O)

Stand facing the wall and place your hands on the wall at shoulder height. Perform a push-up, keeping your body straight and engaging your chest, shoulders, and triceps. Repeat for 10-12 repetitions. This exercise targets the chest, shoulders, and triceps.

The advanced version involves holding one arm behind the back and working with the opposite arm. Alternate supporting arm and repeat the exercise.

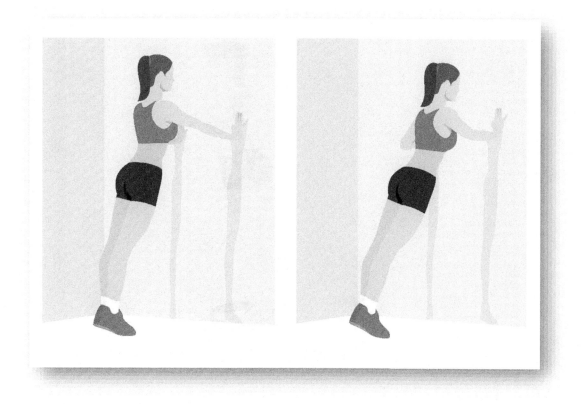

WALL LEG CIRCLES   (EXERCISE P)

This is a lower body exercise that targets the glutes and hip flexors. To perform this exercise, stand facing a wall with your hands at shoulder height on the wall. Next, lift one leg off the floor and draw circles with your foot in the opposite direction. Repeat the movement for 10 to 12 repetitions on each leg.

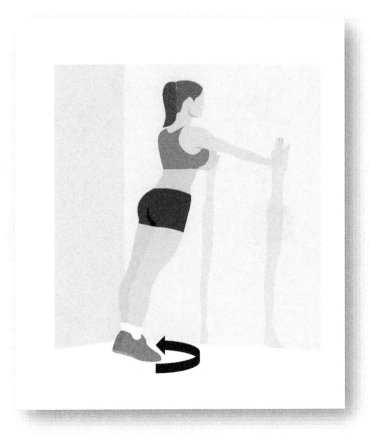

WALL SIDE KEG SWINGS   (EXERCISE K)

Stand sideways to the wall and rest one hand on the wall for balance. Swing one leg, opposite the supported hand, toward the wall and outward while keeping the muscle active and in control of the leg. Then switch legs. Repeat for 10 to 12 repetitions.

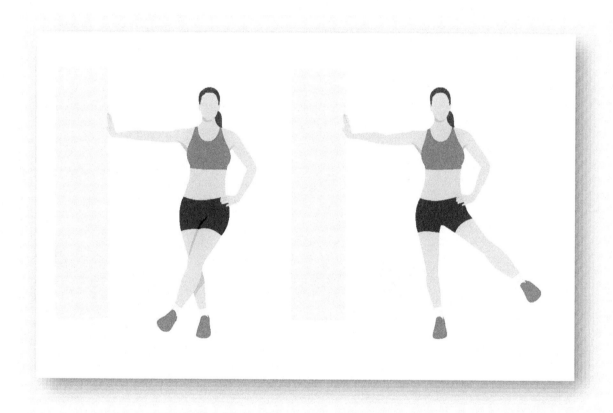

WALL BICYCLE CRUNCHES   (EXERCISE M)

Lie on your back with your legs up the wall, knees bent and feet flat against the wall. Bring one elbow towards the opposite knee, twisting your torso and contracting your abs. Repeat on the other side and continue alternating for 10-12 repetitions. This exercise targets your abs and oblique muscles. (see page 34)

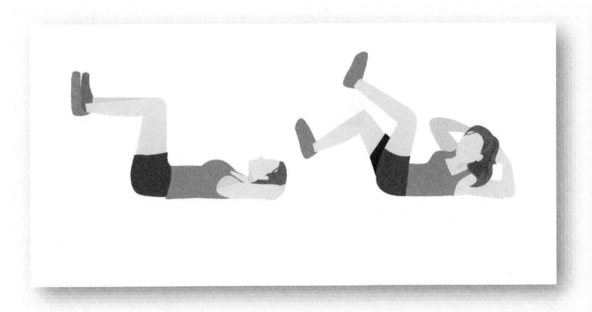

WALL BRIDGE   (EXERCISE Q)

Lie on your back with your feet on the wall and your knees bent. Lift your hips towards the ceiling, contracting your glutes and hamstrings. Lower back down and repeat for 10-12 repetitions. This exercise targets your glutes and hamstrings.(see page 30)

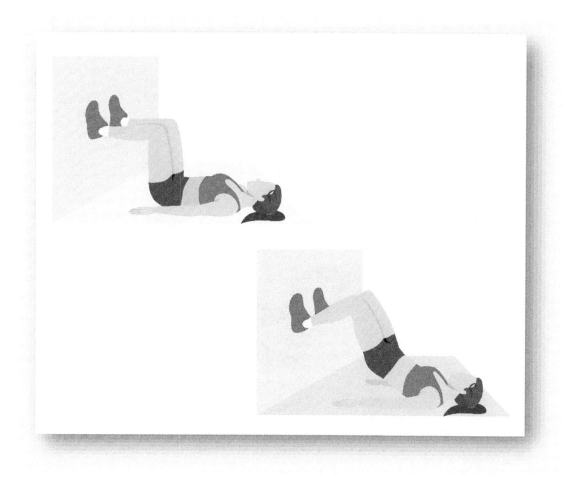

WALL ABDOMINAL CRUNCH   (EXERCISE E)

Lie on your back with your legs against the wall and your hands behind your head. Bring your torso closer to your knees, engaging your abs. Lower yourself down and repeat for 10 to 12 repetitions. The movement does not need to be large and should come mainly from contracting the abdominals. (see page 29)

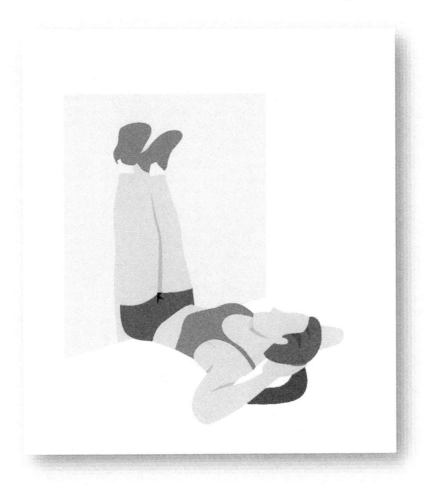

WALL PIKE   (EXERCISE R)

Start in a plank position with your feet against the wall and your hands on the ground. Lift your hips up towards the ceiling, feeling a stretch in your hamstrings. Lower back down and repeat for 10-12 repetitions. (see page 44)

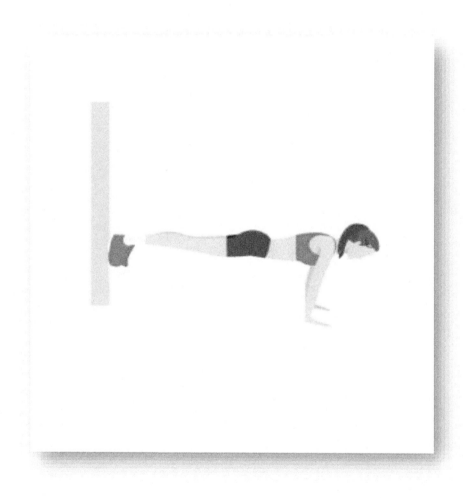

30-DAY Flex & ABS Routine CHART - WEEK 1

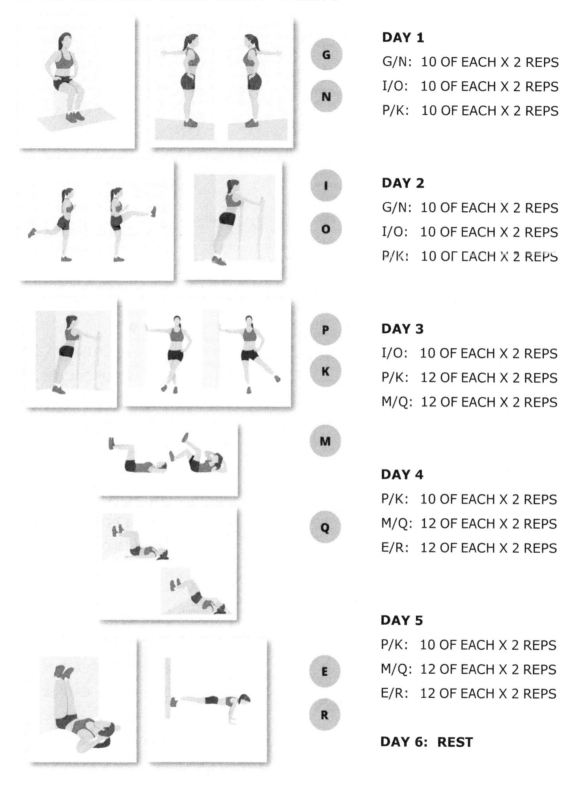

DAY 1

G/N: 10 OF EACH X 2 REPS

I/O: 10 OF EACH X 2 REPS

P/K: 10 OF EACH X 2 REPS

DAY 2

G/N: 10 OF EACH X 2 REPS

I/O: 10 OF EACH X 2 REPS

P/K: 10 OF EACH X 2 REPS

DAY 3

I/O: 10 OF EACH X 2 REPS

P/K: 12 OF EACH X 2 REPS

M/Q: 12 OF EACH X 2 REPS

DAY 4

P/K: 10 OF EACH X 2 REPS

M/Q: 12 OF EACH X 2 REPS

E/R: 12 OF EACH X 2 REPS

DAY 5

P/K: 10 OF EACH X 2 REPS

M/Q: 12 OF EACH X 2 REPS

E/R: 12 OF EACH X 2 REPS

DAY 6: REST

30-DAY Flex & ABS Routine CHART - WEEK 2

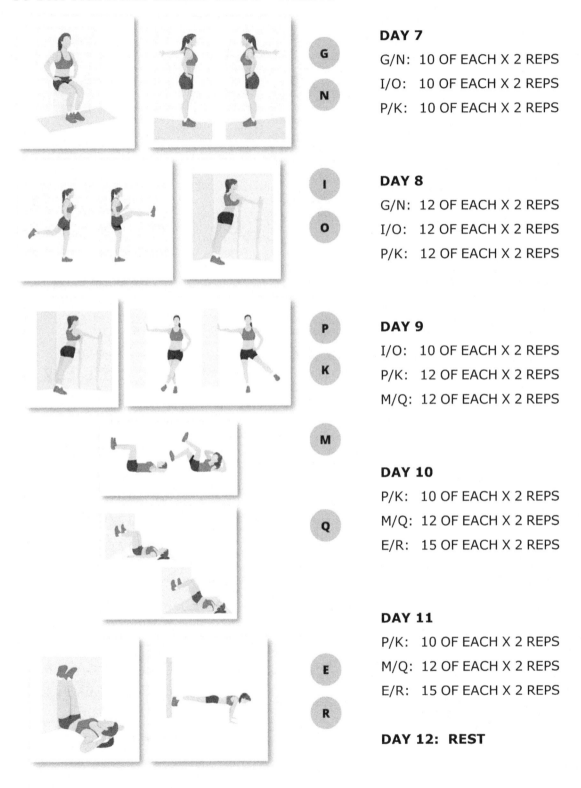

DAY 7

G/N: 10 OF EACH X 2 REPS

I/O: 10 OF EACH X 2 REPS

P/K: 10 OF EACH X 2 REPS

DAY 8

G/N: 12 OF EACH X 2 REPS

I/O: 12 OF EACH X 2 REPS

P/K: 12 OF EACH X 2 REPS

DAY 9

I/O: 10 OF EACH X 2 REPS

P/K: 12 OF EACH X 2 REPS

M/Q: 12 OF EACH X 2 REPS

DAY 10

P/K: 10 OF EACH X 2 REPS

M/Q: 12 OF EACH X 2 REPS

E/R: 15 OF EACH X 2 REPS

DAY 11

P/K: 10 OF EACH X 2 REPS

M/Q: 12 OF EACH X 2 REPS

E/R: 15 OF EACH X 2 REPS

DAY 12: REST

30-DAY Flex & ABS Routine CHART - WEEK 3

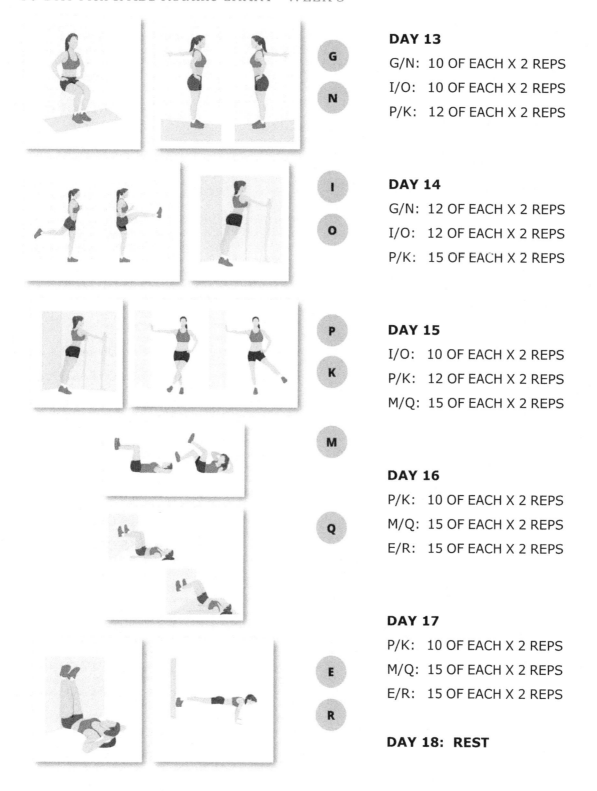

DAY 13

G/N: 10 OF EACH X 2 REPS

I/O: 10 OF EACH X 2 REPS

P/K: 12 OF EACH X 2 REPS

DAY 14

G/N: 12 OF EACH X 2 REPS

I/O: 12 OF EACH X 2 REPS

P/K: 15 OF EACH X 2 REPS

DAY 15

I/O: 10 OF EACH X 2 REPS

P/K: 12 OF EACH X 2 REPS

M/Q: 15 OF EACH X 2 REPS

DAY 16

P/K: 10 OF EACH X 2 REPS

M/Q: 15 OF EACH X 2 REPS

E/R: 15 OF EACH X 2 REPS

DAY 17

P/K: 10 OF EACH X 2 REPS

M/Q: 15 OF EACH X 2 REPS

E/R: 15 OF EACH X 2 REPS

DAY 18: REST

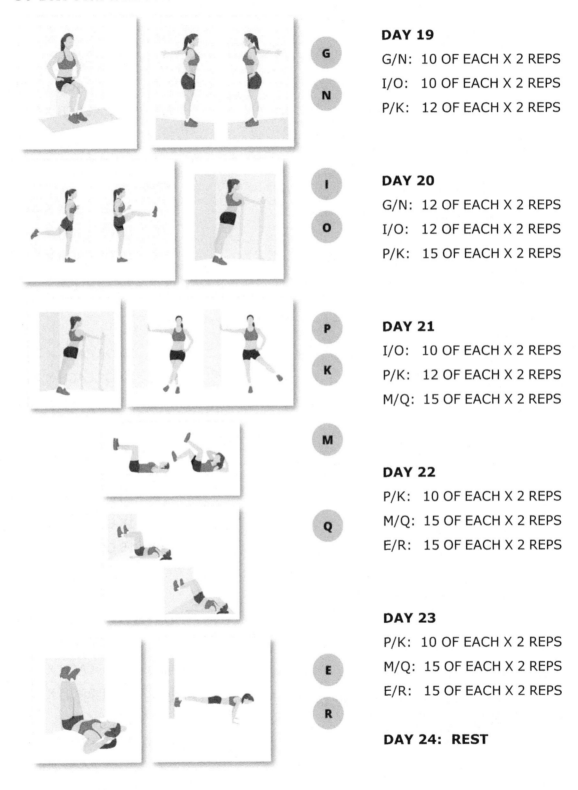

DAY 19

G/N: 10 OF EACH X 2 REPS

I/O: 10 OF EACH X 2 REPS

P/K: 12 OF EACH X 2 REPS

DAY 20

G/N: 12 OF EACH X 2 REPS

I/O: 12 OF EACH X 2 REPS

P/K: 15 OF EACH X 2 REPS

DAY 21

I/O: 10 OF EACH X 2 REPS

P/K: 12 OF EACH X 2 REPS

M/Q: 15 OF EACH X 2 REPS

DAY 22

P/K: 10 OF EACH X 2 REPS

M/Q: 15 OF EACH X 2 REPS

E/R: 15 OF EACH X 2 REPS

DAY 23

P/K: 10 OF EACH X 2 REPS

M/Q: 15 OF EACH X 2 REPS

E/R: 15 OF EACH X 2 REPS

DAY 24: REST

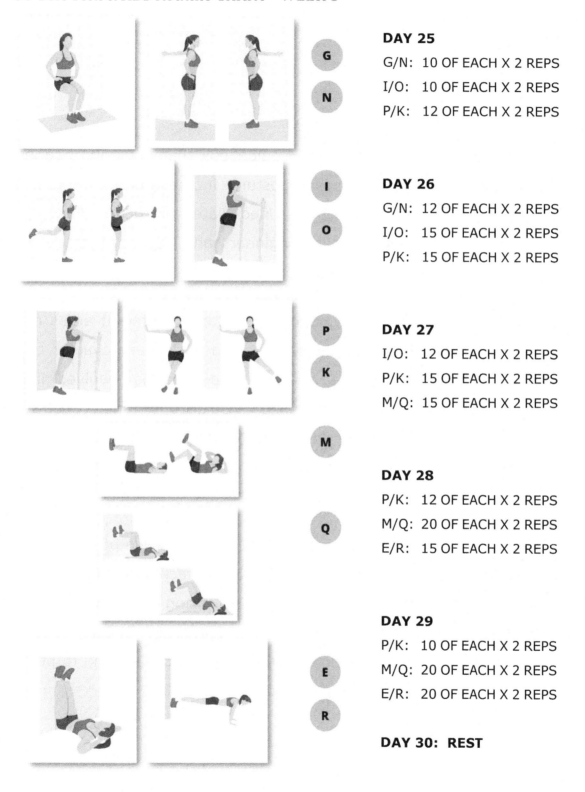

DAY 25

G/N: 10 OF EACH X 2 REPS

I/O: 10 OF EACH X 2 REPS

P/K: 12 OF EACH X 2 REPS

DAY 26

G/N: 12 OF EACH X 2 REPS

I/O: 15 OF EACH X 2 REPS

P/K: 15 OF EACH X 2 REPS

DAY 27

I/O: 12 OF EACH X 2 REPS

P/K: 15 OF EACH X 2 REPS

M/Q: 15 OF EACH X 2 REPS

DAY 28

P/K: 12 OF EACH X 2 REPS

M/Q: 20 OF EACH X 2 REPS

E/R: 15 OF EACH X 2 REPS

DAY 29

P/K: 10 OF EACH X 2 REPS

M/Q: 20 OF EACH X 2 REPS

E/R: 20 OF EACH X 2 REPS

DAY 30: REST

CONCLUSION

Wall Pilates is a comprehensive guidebook that presents a series of exercises designed to improve posture, increase core strength, and enhance flexibility. Written by certified Pilates instructor Ellie Herman, the book is suitable for both beginners and advanced practitioners looking to deepen their practice.

The book is divided into chapters that target different areas of the body, including the arms, legs, core, and back. Each chapter begins with an overview of the anatomy and muscles involved in the exercises, followed by detailed instructions and illustrations demonstrating the proper form and technique. The exercises range from simple stretches and breathing exercises to more challenging movements that require strength, balance, and coordination.

One of the unique features of Wall Pilates is its use of the wall as a prop for many of the exercises. This allows practitioners to use gravity and resistance to their advantage, increasing the intensity of the workout without adding strain to the joints. Additionally, the wall provides support for movements that may be challenging to perform on the mat, such as inversions and handstands.

Another strength of Wall Pilates is its emphasis on mindfulness and breath awareness. Each exercise is accompanied by guidance on breathing techniques that help to deepen the stretch, increase oxygen flow, and promote relaxation. The emphasis on mindfulness also helps practitioners to develop a greater awareness of their body and movement patterns, improving overall body awareness and posture.

Overall, Wall Pilates is a valuable resource for anyone looking to improve their physical health and fitness. The exercises are challenging yet accessible, and the clear instructions and illustrations make it easy to follow along. The use of the wall as a prop adds a unique element to the workout, and the emphasis on mindfulness and breath awareness promotes a deeper connection between the body and mind. Whether you are a beginner or an experienced practitioner, Wall Pilates is a must-read for anyone looking to enhance their Pilates practice.

Made in the USA
Monee, IL
31 May 2023